PCOS Book I
Beating PCOS
Guide

A Guide To An Insulin Resistance Diet That Works For Every Woman

By: Anna Gracey

ISBN-13: 978-1484045251

TABLE OF CONTENTS

Publishers Notes

BLUE SHIFT PUBLISHING LLC

Disclaimer

This publication is intended to provide helpful and informative material. It is not intended to diagnose, treat, cure, or prevent any health problem or condition, nor is intended to replace the advice of a physician. No action should be taken solely on the contents of this book. Always consult your physician or qualified health-care professional on any matters regarding your health and before adopting any suggestions in this book or drawing inferences from it.

The author and publisher specifically disclaim all responsibility for any liability, loss or risk, personal or otherwise, which is incurred as a consequence, directly or indirectly, from the use or application of any contents of this book.

Any and all product names referenced within this book are the trademarks of their respective owners. None of these owners have sponsored, authorized, endorsed, or approved this book.

Always read all information provided by the manufacturers' product labels before using their products. The author and publisher are not responsible for claims made by manufacturers.

The statements made in this book have not been evaluated by the Food and Drug Administration.

Blue Shift Publishing LLC

7950 NW 53rd Street

Miami,

FL 33166

PCOS Book For Women

Paperback Edition 2013

BLUE SHIFT PUBLISHING PRESS is a trademark of Blue Shift Publishing LLC.

For information about special discounts for bulk purchases, please contact Blue Shift Publishing Sales Department at 646-312-7900 or publishing@blueshiftpublishing.com

Designed by Colin WF Scott

Manufactured in the United States of America

Dedication

I want to dedicate this book to every woman that suffers and hass suffered from PCOS, there is no cure for PCOS but there are ways to lead a normal life with using a life formula that I have outlined in this book.

CHAPTER 1- UNDERSTANDING PCOS

Polycystic ovary syndrome (PCOS), what is this?

Polycystic ovary syndrome or PCOS is an issue involving the hormones of a woman being unbalanced. It may result in issues with menstruation and difficulty in getting pregnant. PCOS can also result in unwelcomed changes in appearance. If left untreated for a long while, this condition can result in serious health issues like heart disease and diabetes. The symptoms usually start in teenage years and there are treatments that can aid in the control of symptoms and avoid long-term problems.

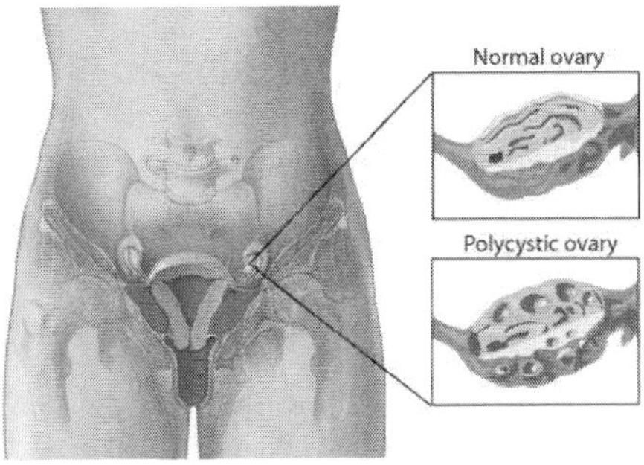

What are the causes of PCOS?

PCOS symptoms result from hormone levels changes. There might be more than one reason for the changes in hormone levels.

This condition tend to be a family tradition, therefore, if other women in the family are experiencing this condition, diabetes or irregular periods, this can be inherited from the father or mother's side of the family.

The role of hormones in PCOS

Hormones are known as chemical messengers that activate a variety of processes which include energy production and growth. Frequently, one hormone's task is simply to signal another hormone's release.

For reasons that are not yet fully understood, the condition of PCOS involves hormones getting out of balance. There will be one change in hormone that can trigger one other change and this change can occur again. For instance, sex hormones may become imbalanced; normally, a small amount of masculine sex hormones or androgens are made by the ovaries. In PCOS, little more androgens are created. This might result in the interruption of ovulation, getting acne and growing excess body and facial hair.

What symptoms come with PCOS?

The symptoms usually are not so harsh at first and some persons may experience few while some get a good amount of them. The symptoms that are most common include acne, difficulty losing weight, weight gain, excess body and face hair, scalp hair thinning, irregular periods (usually less than nine a year, no periods sometimes, and heavy bleeding), fertility issues and also depression.

Majority of women having this condition may have a small cyst growing on the ovaries. This is the reason it is labeled 'polycystic ovary syndrome.' Although the cysts may not be considered harmful, it can result in hormone imbalances.

How is PCOS treated?

Some very effective PCOS treatments include regular exercise, weight control and healthy foods. Medicines that are designed to balance out hormones can be used also. Treating the condition can result in the decrease of unpleasant symptoms and aid in the prevention of health problems that are long-term.

Foods that are healthy for the heart as well as exercise to manage PCOS can aid in lowering cholesterol and blood pressure and lessen the danger of diabetes and also heart disease. These can also help the individual in losing weight if there is a need to.

A diet that is considered heart-healthy generally has a lot of whole grains, beans, nuts, fruits and vegetables. This diet also is very low in foods that are rich in saturated fats like fried foods, cheeses and meats. If an individual has problems with blood sugar, attempts should be made to eat the same level of carbohydrate for every meal. A licensed dietician can aid the individual in making an ideal meal plan.

Smokers tend to have a higher level androgen which might trigger PCOS symptoms and smoking usually increase heart disease risks.

Some medicines may also be prescribed by a doctor like:

Metformin (a medicine for diabetes) – This can aid in the restoration of normal menstrual cycles as well as fertility.

Birth control pills – These help to make periods regular and normal and may lessen symptoms like acne and unwelcomed facial hair. There are other medicines like spironolactone that lower the androgen levels that are generally used with the birth control pills, but these are not advised to be used if the individual is trying to conceive.

Fertility medicines – These are usually for persons who are making attempts to become pregnant.

Prescribed as well as over-the-counter medicines might help with skin issues.

Chapter 2- Negative Effects of Living with PCOS

There are very unpleasant symptoms that come with this condition. Among these is, in addition to irregular menstrual cycles, oily skin, acne, too much body hair, Type 2 diabetes, obesity, high blood pressure and elevated cholesterol level, sleep apnea, infertility as well as thinning hair (sometimes balding that is similar to that of males). The uterus lining also becomes particularly thick because of the absence of regular periods. In addition, when a period eventually occurs, it can be unusually heavy and may come with uncomfortable cramping.

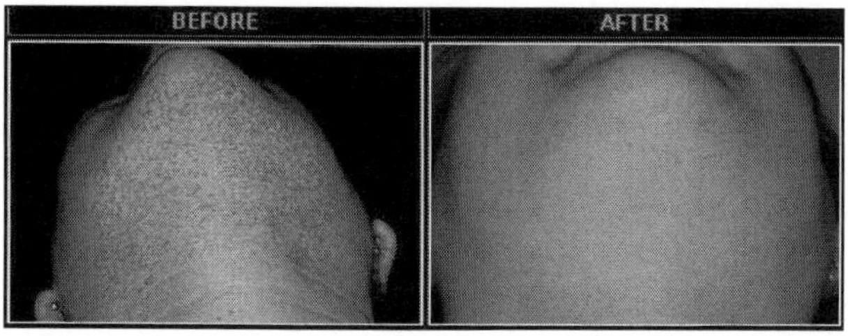

If the symptoms are untreated, it might make the matter worse. However, the treatments come with their own risks. Frequently, women who have no desire to become pregnant will be treated with birth control pills to allow the regulation of menstrual cycles. Side effects of some birth control pills include stroke, nausea, blood clots, insomnia, weight fluctuations, fever, and some amount of moodiness. Under normal circumstances, some women experience a few of these side effects also.

Getting Pregnant Despite Higher Rate of Infertility with PCOS – The Most Pressing Question

If attempts are being made for some time now to get pregnant to no avail, the first thought usually is that infertility is involved. Fertility is very important. The fact is though, that majority of couples require a minimum of six to twelve months to conceive, even when circumstances are good. Also, a lot of women who experience PCOS are successful in getting pregnant.

However, in addition to the stress involved in trying to get pregnant and ovulation issues which may come with PCOS, it may even take longer sometimes. Therefore to become pregnant, there are some important things that need to be done.

Ovulation: The woman is required to be releasing eggs from the ovaries and this is better if it is done regularly. A menstrual period that is regular usually indicates proper ovulation. When the menstrual cycles are lengthy, this could mean that ovulation is infrequent.

Women that have PCOS, however, do not get regular cycles and as a result ovulation does not occur regularly. This will result in the difficulty of getting the fertile time correct. It is often reported that women have menstruation that occur for four weeks and up to twenty weeks. They do not know whether or not ovulation is taking place. At this point, some blood tests are usually done to find out for sure.

Fallopian tubes: These are required to be open (not blocked). This is referred to by doctors as Patent fallopian tubes. They are capable of picking up the egg that is released. The egg fertilization by the sperm from the partner happens in the outside third of the fallopian tube.

CHAPTER 3- PREGNANCY WITH PCOS

If pregnancy occurs while having PCOS, the woman can experience health issues that are greater when compared the regular population. The problems include high blood pressure that is induced by pregnancy, gestational diabetes, premature delivery and miscarriage. Research has also found that health problems like macrosomia (babies born larger than 4,500 grams), pre-eclampsia, as well as clotting factors occurring in women who are pregnant and have PCOS.

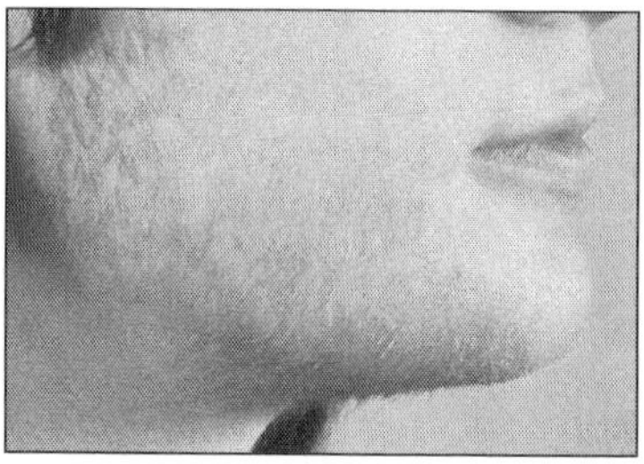

Gestational Diabetes

Although the female may have never had problems with diabetes before, blood sugar levels can escalate during pregnancy. This is called gestational diabetes. Approximately four percent of pregnant women worldwide are affected by this complication. Research shows that women that were diagnosed with gestational diabetes during pregnancy are known to have more elevated PCOS prevalence when screened. It is believed that the risk is greater among women who are obese and that need ovulation induction for conceiving to take place.

Pregnancy-induced High Blood Pressure

Any female that have borderline hypertension prior to pregnancy is expected to have more elevated blood pressure during pregnancy, but majority of doctors examine all the patients for issues relating to blood pressure. This should be documented right through the pregnancy.

Insulin Resistance and Miscarriage

For women who are experiencing PCOS and have been able to conceive, they could have a higher possibility of miscarriage when compared to women who do not have this condition. Some researches calculate the miscarriage rate for women having PCOS as forty-five percent, compared to the general fifteen percent average.

Levels of high insulin can essentially result in the increase of blood clotting at the border between the lining of the uterine and placenta, resulting in the insufficiency of the placenta; this is when the placenta fail to supply necessary nutrients to fetus and eliminate toxic wastes. This leads to miscarriage.

Premature Delivery

About thirty to forty percent of EPL (early pregnancy loss) are related to PCOS; EPL is known to be miscarriage that occurs in the first trimester. In majority of cases, there is no identified cause, but, not only defects in the development of the embryo, unfavorable changes in the endometrial function can be a factor. The dysfunction of insulin has been recognized as an EPL risk factor that stands on its own.

Promoting Healthy Pregnancy

Particular steps can be taken to encourage general health which may be helpful also in making sure that there is a healthy pregnancy that is free from complications in the days, months or years to come. The steps include making overall improvement to diet, doing more exercise, cutting down stress levels while balancing the hormone systems as well as getting an adequate and balanced amount of necessary nutraceuticals.

Insulite PCOS System includes the approaches that are required to control PCOS and the Insulin Resistance that is underlying, which may be able to assist in reducing health risks which may occur during a pregnancy.

CHAPTER 4- TREATING PCOS NATURALLY

Supplements

Inosotol, Folic Acid and Vitamin D

Inosotol is also called vitamin B-8 and is proven to reduce the resistance to insulin and improve the symptoms of PCOS in women. Studies have also shown that when inosotol is taken with folic acid, a B vitamin (B-9), there is improvement in ovulatory function as well as raised lipoprotein levels of high density; this is the 'good' kind of protective cholesterol. It has been proven that the combination of folic acid and inosotol worked better when compared to the effect of folic acid by itself to improve the symptoms of PCOS. To prevent defects of the neural tube which can occur in the early part of the pregnancy, women are advised to take a minimum of 400 mg of the folic acid on a daily basis if they are trying to conceive. Vitamin D (along with calcium) is given to women with PCOS to reduce insulin resistance and cut down the symptoms of PCOS.

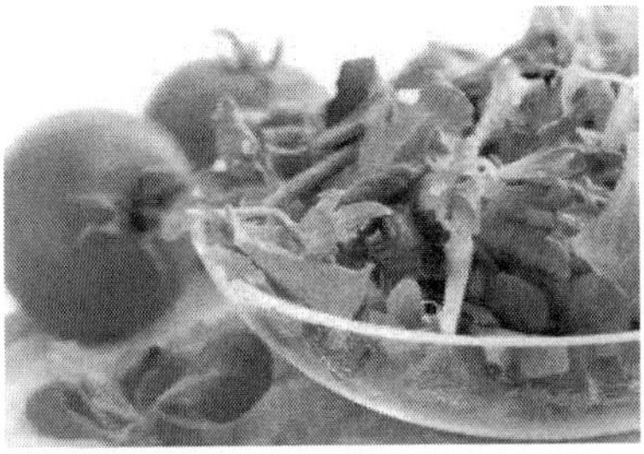

Managing PCOS And Depression

Even though PCOS is not a fatal condition, it is still challenging for thousands of females who experience it. Because it comes with symptoms which include acne, hirsutism (excessive hair growth), infertility, obesity, hair loss, it comes as no surprise that the self-esteem of a woman can be significantly affected by PCOS.

Every woman will experience PCOS differently and not all will have the same level of severity in symptoms or problems relating to infertility. As such, each female with this condition will be affected in different ways. Self-esteem is formed by what one experiences in life and also skills for coping. These are in addition to external aspects like the problems mentioned earlier.

Since testosterone is a principal male hormone, heightened levels can result in symptoms that are known to be masculine, such as baldness, acne, hair growing on the stomach, chest or face. The condition of high androgen in PCOS also results in irregular periods. Because of the masculine traits that develop, it is usual for several women having this syndrome to feel unfeminine or masculine. This can greatly affect her self-esteem.

The main difficulty in treating PCOS symptoms is that these are derived from hormonal imbalances. Traditional medication or treatment routines for conditions such as hair loss or acne might not have any effect if the hormonal abnormalities are not being addressed as well.

Infertility

A woman's self-esteem as well as identity can be significantly affected if she is experiencing the condition of infertility. Society makes it difficult for these women to feel feminine if they are not able to get pregnant and as a result, a woman's personal perception can be altered. When this is added to the rest of symptoms that come with PCOS, it is no wonder why self-doubt and depression are prevalent in women having this condition.

Having to go through treatment for infertility and having the private life exposed can cause stress on a marriage. This further affects the self-esteem. The woman might feel she is being blamed or she might harbor guilt feelings, believing that the condition and treatment is totally her fault.

Weight

Women who have PCOS generally struggle with their weight. The androgen levels that are elevated may result in insulin resistance as well as weight gain, particularly around the waist and abdomen. In addition, women who have PCOS experience an exceptionally hard time getting rid of the weight, even if she is making every effort to lose it.

It is suggested that women experiencing this really challenging time with their weight, should not give up and try harder. If required, consult a registered dietician and/or an exercise trainer to help in the quest to lose some weight.

CHAPTER 5- THE COMPLETE PCOS DIET PLAN

GI or glycemic index is known as the most ideal tool that is available to place food that are rich in carbohydrate in classes in accordance to their capabilities of elevating the levels of blood sugar when consumed. The foods that are high on the index (above 70) can cause blood sugar levels to rapidly increase and at the same time set off a large amount of insulin release. Low-GI foods (below 55) will give slow increase in the levels of blood sugar and this comes with smaller insulin release from the body's pancreas.

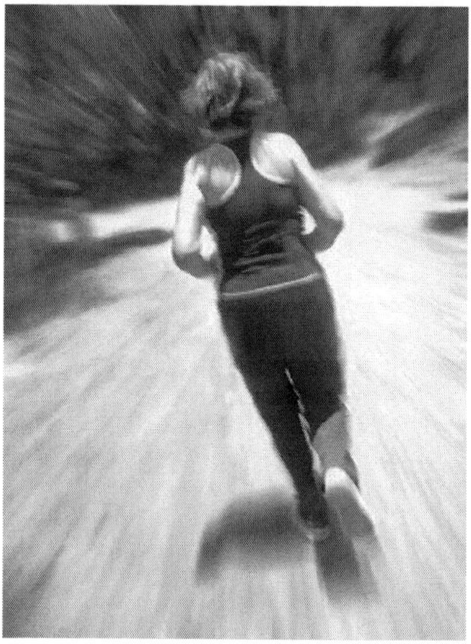

On the foods that contain carbohydrates are known to have GI as it is not possible to calculate the GI of any food that has a lot of fat like butter or oil, foods that are protein-rich, like eggs and meat, or any food that do not have adequate levels of carbohydrates like lettuce or broccoli.

Low GI Diet and Insulin Resistance

Foods having lower GI may be particularly useful for women that have PCOS. Because of the slow rise in the levels of blood sugar, the consumption of these foods usually results in lower insulin levels. Researchers have found that the women that fall in the diet group having low GI had considerably better improvements in insulin sensitivity and almost all (ninety-five percent) of them benefitted as well from a menstrual cycle that was improved.

Low GI Foods

If the decision is made to adopt a diet that is low in GI to be better able to manage the PCOS, carbohydrates that have high GI have to be eliminated first, like fried, boiled or mashed potatoes, breakfast cereals that have been processed, whole grain or white bread, dates, jelly beans and white rice.

CHAPTER 6- TOP TEN MUST EAT INGREDIENTS FOR YOUR PCOS DIET – WHAT I CALL SUPERFOODS

Romaine Lettuce

The chromium that is found in romaine lettuce aids in fighting insulin resistance.

Lettuce has low calories and may be used as the base for delectable and light salads. This type of lettuce provides lots of health-related benefits, especially for women who experience the negative symptoms of PCOS. Romaine lettuce is also supercharged with several essential nutrients like chromium. This is an element of the GTF (glucose tolerance factor) which aids in maintaining regular levels of blood sugar by making the insulin to be more efficient. This reduces insulin resistance that frequently comes with PCOS. In addition, chromium enhances weight loss because of its capability of helping to control cravings and the fat that is in the blood as well as reduce hunger.

Turnip Greens

Turnip plant leaves are called turnip greens. This is an old-time vegetable which was initially grown approximately 4,000 years in the past in Near East. It comes from the plant genus known as Brassica that includes a lot of other plants that promotes health like collards, cabbage and broccoli. These vegetables are exceptionally low in calories but have a lot of nutrients that promote weight loss and fight PCOS. These include calcium and vitamin C. In addition, the calcium found in the turnip greens is available for use by the body as a result of the oxalic acid that appears in low levels in these turnips. This oxalic acid that is prevalent in several other green foods is proven to hinder calcium absorption.

Barley

Women that have PCOS will find barley highly beneficial. In addition to being low in calories, it has the rating that is the lowest on the glycemic index when compared with all the common grains. The body rapidly breaks down the grains having high ratings on the GI, resulting in a quick and large increase in the levels of blood glucose. This in turn activates the releasing of larger insulin amounts from the pancreas. The body requires a particular level of insulin, but when the levels are too high, this can result in the body resisting insulin and also obesity. This can make the PCOS symptoms to worsen. On the other hand, carbs having low GI like barley generally take a considerably longer time to be digested and result in a slow, small rise in the levels of insulin and blood glucose. Also, these low-GI foods decrease craving.

Cinnamon

There are some exceptional benefits that come with cinnamon which may aid in increasing the sensitivity to insulin and therefore treat PCOS and also obesity. Only ½ teaspoon of this cinnamon daily has proven to be quite effective in normalizing the levels of blood sugar and cut down food cravings. The primary component of cinnamon is hydroxychalcone that is believed to promote insulin effect. Cinnamon also seems to stop blood sugar hikes after a meal by slowing down the GER (gastric emptying rate). This means that the stomach will retain the food longer.

Crimini Mushrooms

The crimini mushrooms are known to be an ideal functional provision for persons that suffer from the condition of PCOS. These are good B vitamins sources that have low calories, especially of B-2 vitamin which is necessary for metabolism and regular thyroid and which may therefore aid in the reduction of excess weight of the body. They are high also in B-3 vitamin which assists in keeping blood sugar balanced. These mushrooms can be eaten either cooked or raw. When they are served raw, they can be sprinkled with some lemon juice to stop them from becoming dark brown in color.

Broccoli

Broccoli is a green crunchy vegetable that is believed to be the most ideal food for women who have PCOS. Calorie content is low and there is less than one percent of fat. It also has low GI rating. Broccoli is a great source of calcium that is free of dairy. To optimize on the health benefits of broccoli, the plants that are organically grown should be chosen as these are generally more filled with nutrients and have less harmful substances. Slightly steamed or raw broccoli is also more beneficial.

Salmon

Salmon is known as a high vitamin D source in any diet. PCOS have reported vitamin D levels that are low and resulting in problems such as weight gain, infertility, as well as insulin resistance. Additionally, salmon is high in magnesium, vitamins B-6 and B-3. These components are proven to aid in the maintenance of normal levels of blood sugar, fertility and hormonal balance. Select wild salmon over the farm-fresh one when purchasing salmon. However, it is advised that salmon should only be consumed in moderation, whatever the choice may be as high salmon consumption (over two times per week) may put persons at risk of large amounts of pesticides and mercury that are found in some fish. Women who desire and are making attempts at conceiving should be particularly careful because the toxins in this fish could damage fetus' neurological development.

Wheat Germ

One of the most ideal foods for fighting PCOS is wheat germ. It offers a concentrated vitamin B-6 source or pyridoxine; this along with a small amount of wheat germ can provide seventy-five percent of the daily consumption that is recommended for this essential vitamin. When wheat germ is added to cereals, breads, milk shakes, pancakes or muesli, it turn out to be a nutritional but unnoticed addition. It is an excellent supply of other B-vitamins and also zinc. It also has a lot of magnesium. It should be importantly noted when wheat germ is being stored, that it can become rancid real fast and this is as a result of the unsaturated fat that it contains. To get the most from it, store it in a dry, cool place in container that is sealed and keep it away from sun exposure.

Sunflower Seeds

There are several benefits to be gained from sunflower seeds. First of all, they have lot of calories but this not a reason to stay away from sunflower seeds. What is required is for them to be consumed in moderation to get optimum health benefits. The several nutrients contained in sunflower seeds help to fight the symptoms that come with PCOS. These nutrients include riboflavin or vitamin B-2 as well as pyridoxine (vitamin B-6), an exceptional combination of nutrient that is great against the symptoms of PCOS. Only one cup of sunflower seed can provide 31% of what is recommended as daily intake of vitamin B-6. Sunflower seeds also have loads of magnesium and zinc which are two necessary minerals for fighting PCOS.

Kale

Known as a nutritional base, kale has several minerals and vitamins and is known as an ideal plant-based calcium source. Calcium is essential for egg maturation and the development of follicle inside the ovaries. The leaves of the kale which are tender may be eaten uncooked, for instance, as an iceberg lettuce substitute in salads. It can be transformed also in a heart-healthy dish when the leaves are sautéed and mixed with chopped up onions, a little bit of some extra virgin olive oil and crush garlic. When purchasing kale, it is recommended that the one that is grown organically is selected as it is known that kale that is conventionally grown has more chemical and pesticide content when compared to other vegetables.

OTHER GREAT FOODS THAT ARE RECOMMENDED

Sesame Seeds

Sesame seeds have a whole lot of nutrients which are proven as being especially beneficial for women who have PCOS. The small seeds are excellent vitamin B-6 source and only half of a cup can provide over a quarter of what is recommended to be consumed each day. In addition, they offer great source of calcium that is plant-based, magnesium and some fatty acids that offer health benefits. Zinc is also included in sesame seeds and these are available all year round. They add a tasty and nutty flavor as well as a little crunch to several Asian dishes.

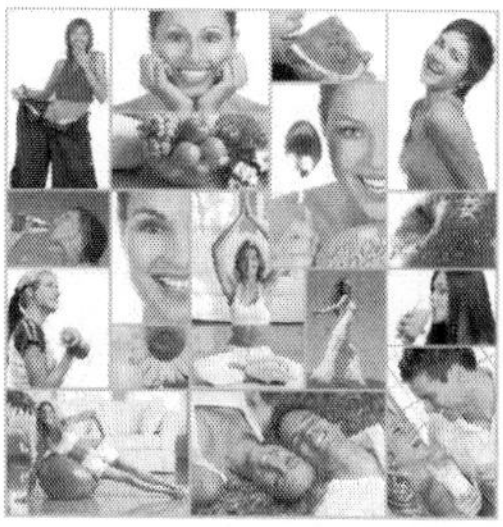

Chicken Breast

If concern exists about excess weight and PCOS, an ideal food that should be added to shopping lists is chicken breast. This offers great source of protein but has very low carbohydrate and fat content. Other nutrients that is offered in chicken breast include vitamins B-3 and B-6. The vitamin B-3 can be especially useful for persons whose waistline is expanding and which is associated with insulin resistance. The vitamin B-6 is vital for maintaining balance of hormones as well as fertility.

Poppy Seeds

Poppy seeds can be sprinkled on the top of a favorite dish. They have loads of healthy advantages which include the decreased danger of symptoms of PCOS. Although they are small in size, poppy seeds have a lot of calcium, B vitamins, zinc and magnesium. All of these components are vital for the prevention as well as the treatment of PCOS symptoms.

Tuna

Tuna is great for adding to the diet for women who are overweight and desire to fight against PCOS by getting rid of excess weight. In each tuna water-packed container there are nearly thirty-three grams of protein with no carbohydrates or fat involved. Protein contains exceptionally elevated thermogenic effect (twenty to thirty percent), which indicates that a considerably amount of the calories that is offered by a food that is rich in protein, like tuna, is burnt by the body when the food is being broken down and digested.

In addition, vitamin D and B vitamins are contained in tuna and these are essential for women having PCOS. However, in the process of adding tuna to any diet, it must be kept in mind that it should be eaten in moderation. If it is consumed too frequently or in amounts that are too high, persons may be exposed to particular toxins like mercury. The recommended serving size for tuna is six or less. Breastfeeding and pregnant women especially should be especially cautious as the toxins that are in fish may be exceptionally dangerous to newborn babies and fetuses.

Chapter 7- Top Ten Things That You Must Do To Beat PCOS

Reduce Calories Intake, Particularly Evening Time

High intake of energy is known to be linked with increased threat of PCOS, mostly as it is capable of contributing to overweight and obesity development. For weight loss, a deficit of calorie has to be created, either by the reduction of the intake of calorie from foods in order for the body to be forced to pull on energy reserves (like fat stored in the body) or when physical activity is increased. Methods of cooking which utilize little fat (like roasting or steaming vegetables without the use of oil) are able to significantly help in the reduction of calorie intake. Research has also found that a diet that restricts calories may help in normalizing hormones, treat infertility and induce ovulation.

Effective weight loss aids in fighting PCOS symptoms

Majority of health professionals suggest that 3,500-7,000 caloric deficit is created each week for successful and healthy weight loss. Deficit that is over 7,000-10,500 calories for a week (extreme deficit) can thwart bodily functions as well as lead to abnormalities in heart beat and this can be deadly.

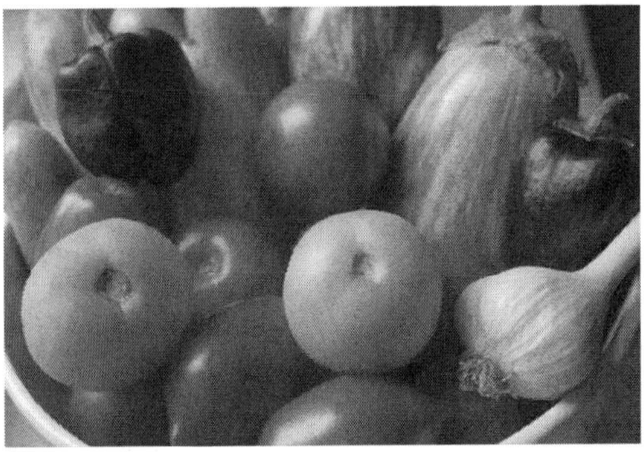

In addition, if calories are excessively cut, it might be end up being counterproductive to efforts to lose weight, as diets which are very low in the content of calories boost enzymes to be stored in the body and reduce the fat-burning enzyme activity. Also, excessive cutting of calories may cause the acceleration of loss of muscle mass (lean) and reduce thyroid hormone output, resulting in a reduction of metabolic rate. This will cause a fewer amount of calories to be burned during the day.

Women who are overweight must also be attentive to when calorie is consumed on a daily basis. It is usually suggested that calories are spread out during the day by eating five to six small meals. When this is done, metabolism will remain humming and there will be reduced starch and sweets cravings, which are frequent among women that have PCOS. The biggest meal each day must be breakfast as this will greatly help in getting the metabolism started and more fat will be burned during the day.

Select Low-GI Carbs

The body quickly breaks down carbs that are rated high on the GI rating and result in a quick and great increase in the levels of blood glucose, which also triggers pancreas to emit insulin of large amounts. Insulin is essential for the body to be capable of using glucose for the purpose of energy, but too much insulin may result in the resistance of insulin as well obesity, which might make the symptoms of PCOS worse. In contrast, carbs having low GI, which usually take a longer time to digest, result in only a slow and small rise in the levels of insulin and blood glucose. Also, these foods cut down cravings, which may cause weight gain, because they offer a steady and slow energy supply. Majority of fruits, legumes and vegetables that are non-starchy have low GI score while a lot of refined foods that are rich in carbohydrate have high rating on the GI.

Consume Plenty B vitamins

The symptoms of PCOS may be alleviated with B vitamins, particularly B-6, B-5, B-3, and B2. Energy is converted from carbohydrates, protein and dietary fat with the help of vitamin B-2. The vitamin B3 aids in maintaining the normal levels of blood sugar. Vitamins B-5 can assist in weight loss because of its capability to manage the metabolism of fat. The B-6 is essential for maintaining balance of hormones and fertility. In addition, it is required for adequate absorption of important zinc into the intestines. The vitamins B-6, B-2 and B-3 are vital for normal metabolism and thyroid function, and can therefore aid in the reduction of extra body weight.

Ensure an Adequate Intake of Vitamin D and Calcium

Several studies conclude that calcium is probably effective in treating PCOS. The calcium is essential for the maturation of egg as well as follicle development which occur in the ovaries. The absorption of calcium from food that is in the intestine is enhanced by vitamin D. In addition, vitamin D of low levels is related to issues relating to PCOS, which include weight gain, resistance to insulin and infertility.

Eat Foods High in Zinc

The job of the mineral zinc is to fight obesity and acne which are frequent with PCOS.

Research finds that zinc can get rid of the symptoms of acne, particularly if there is a lack of this essential mineral. In addition, some researchers find that the supplementation of zinc can have as much impact as treating the acne with traditional antibiotics. The zinc properties that fight acne are thought of as resulting from its capability to decrease inflammation, reduce the production sebum on the skin's surface and destroy the bacteria that is linked with acne. Zinc is also important in the synthesis of protein and in the formation of collagen. The two of them are essential for getting and keeping healthy skin.

The supplementations of this element to subjects that are deficient in zinc are known to heighten leptin circulation levels. When leptin levels are not sufficient, this is believed to result in food cravings as well as overeating. Both actions can contribute to PCOS-associated obesity.

Consume Plenty Foods Containing Magnesium

There is research that suggests that a strong association exist between the deficiencies in magnesium as well as insulin resistance that is linked with PCOS. Adequate glucose utilization as well as insulin signaling requires magnesium. Both of these are damaged in persons having insulin resistance. It seems like magnesium is the most popular micronutrient that is found to be lacking in individuals that are resistant to insulin as well as diabetic patients.

Calcium and magnesium works synergistically together. An adequate ratio of these two minerals (a ratio of 2:1 calcium to magnesium is usually recommended), is required for them to optimally work. Mild magnesium deficiency is relatively common among women that live in countries in the Western region, where the consumption of processed foods is prevalent, because processing considerably decrease magnesium in food contents. In addition, intensive farming that is practiced in several Western countries depletes the magnesium in the soil, and thus decreasing the content of magnesium of plants that grow in the soil.

Eat Foods Containing Chromium

Chromium is an element of GTF or glucose tolerance factor which aids in maintaining regular levels of blood glucose by making the insulin to be more effective. This will battle against insulin resistance that is frequently linked with PCOS. In addition, chromium enhances weight loss because of its capability to assist in controlling cravings, control fat found in the blood and reduce hunger.

Chromium deficiencies are frequent among persons that eat plenty processed foods, because processing takes away the content of chromium from foods. Also, persons who consume a lot of tea, sugar or coffee have an increased danger of being chromium deficient. Chromium sources that are considered efficient include potatoes, tomatoes, whole grains, onions and romaine lettuce. To optimize the health benefits of these foods, they should be combined with foods that are rich in vitamin C; this increases chromium absorption.

Think About Eating Licorice Root

Licorice has glycyrrhizin content that is known to considerably cut down plasma testosterone. This is great revelation for persons that have PCOS with elevated levels of testosterone, hirsutism or acne. If the intention is to consume the licorice to try to make PCOS stay within the level of control, bear in mind that when licorice is consumed frequently in large quantities, this can result in high blood pressure, potassium depletion, edema, heart problems, headaches and other health problems.

Chapter 8- My Top Pick Recipes For Women With PCOS

BREAKFAST

Dairy-Free Blueberry Muesli

For 4 servings

Ingredients

1 ½ cups of oats rolled

½ cup chopped walnuts

½ cup chopped dried apples

2 teaspoon Ground cinnamon

2 cups wild blueberries

3 table spoon brown sugar

To serve with Apple juice

Instructions

Heat oven to 325°Fahrenheit or 160°Celsius, gas 3.

In a bowl mix together rolled oats, sugar, and cinnamon. Onto a non-sticking baking tray spread out mixture evenly.

Toast oat combination in oven that is preheated for approximately ten minutes, occasionally stirring. Observe mixture closely when toasting since it can burn quite easily.

Take out of the oven and allow it to cool. Pour in a big bowl and mix in chopped walnuts along with dried apples.

Separate mixture in serving bowls and top with blueberries. This can be served with apple juice.

Muffins for Weight Loss

12 servings of muffins

Ingredients

1 cup oats rolled, soaked in 1 cup skim milk for 1-2 hrs.

½ cup applesauce that is unsweetened

2 egg whites

1 cup skim milk

1 cup flour (whole wheat)

½ cup dark sugar

1 teaspoon baking powder

½ teaspoon baking soda

½ teaspoon salt

1 teaspoon cinnamon

1 cup blueberries

Instructions

Heat oven to 400 degrees Fahrenheit or 200 degrees Celsius, gas mark 6.

Beat together egg whites, a mixture of oat and milk along with applesauce. Put together the ingredients that are in a separate bowl.

Add the liquid ingredients to the dry items and mix up until they are combined do not mix excessively. Blueberries should be folded at this stage.

Once the blueberries are folded, fill up 12 paper muffin cups with the batter to around two thirds full. Then put in oven and bake for about twenty minutes or until it is done.

Oat and Wheat Germ Muesli with Apples

Serves Four (4)

Recipe

1 1/2 cups uncooked or rolled toasted oats

1/2 cup wheat germ

2 teaspoon ground cinnamon

1 1/2 cup diced organic apples

2 tablespoon brown sugar

Serve with yoghurt that is organic and have probiotic bacteria.

Instructions

Oven should be preheated to 325°Farhenheit or 160°Celsius, gas 3.

Combine sugar, oats along with cinnamon in a bowl. Mixture should be spread evenly on a non-stick tray used for baking.

Place toast oat combination in preheated oven for roughly ten (10) minutes, occasionally stir. Observe the toasting mixture closely as it can easily burn.

Take out the mixture from the oven and allow it to cool. Once it cooled pour in a big bowl and mix in wheat germ.

Separate mixture into serving bowls and use as apples and raspberries as toppings. Serve up with yoghurt.

Raspberry Low Glycemic Muffins

Serving of ten (10) muffins

Recipe

1 1/2 cups flour (whole wheat)

1/2 cup flour (soy)

2 teaspoon baking powder

1/3 cup sugar (brown)

2 teaspoon cinnamon

2 egg whites

1 cup milk (soy)

2 Tablespoon canola oil

1 cup raspberries

Instructions

Oven to be preheated to 375°Farhenhit or 190°Celsius, gas mark 5.

Mix ingredients that are dry in a large bowl. Beat together egg whites, the soy milk as well as the canola oil in a different bowl.

Add together the wet ingredients in the dry and mix until blended, try not mix excessively. Fold raspberries.

Fill up 12 muffin paper cups with batter to approximately two thirds. Bake for around 15 – 20 minutes or until the tester toothpick comes out clean.

Original Bircher Muesli

Serve 1

Recipe

1 tablespoon rolled oats

3 tablespoon water

1 tablespoon condensed milk that is sweetened

2 teaspoon lemon juice

1-2 apples include the skin

1 tablespoon hazelnuts or almonds, ground

Instructions

Mix oats and water and keep in the refrigerator overnight. Soaking enhances the dietary value of oats as it permits the enzymes to break down and counteract phytic acid, which is a composite that is able to block the absorption of a lot of minerals in the intestines.

Grate apples and add them collectively with sweetened condensed milk and lemon juice, to the soaked oats. Once this is done ensure that you stir the mixture well.

Shake over with almonds or hazelnuts then serve.

SOUPS AND SALADS

Steamed Asparagus with Sesame Seeds

Recipe

1 tablespoon sesame seeds

2 pounds asparagus

1 tbsp lemon juice

2 tablespoon extra-virgin olive oil

2 teaspoon sesame oil

2 teaspoon fresh grated ginger

Add Salt and freshly ground black pepper to taste

Instructions

Mix sesame seeds in a hot non-stick frying pan until it is golden brown.

Use a small bowl and beat together the sesame oil, lemon juice, ginger, olive oil, salt and pepper.

Set up a steamer with boiling water then add the asparagus, cover and allow to steam until it is tender crisp, this should be around three to five minutes. When asparagus is tender crisp, pour the oil and ginger mixture over it.

Move to a serving platter and shake sesame seeds over the platter.

Carrot and Beet Soup

For a Serving of Four (4)

Recipe

3 average beets, peeled as well as diced

1 tablespoon canola oil

1 cup chopped onion

1 lb diced carrots

1 tablespoon minced fresh ginger

1 clove minced garlic

6 cups stock vegetable

Instructions

Heat up oil in a big saucepan over average heat. Sauté onion until a golden brown colour is seen. Add minced garlic clove and ginger then cook for 2 minutes, frequently stirring.

Put in beets, carrots, and vegetable stock. Turn the heat to low and allow it to simmer while covered until beets and carrots become tender, this should take roughly twenty-five (25) minutes.

In separate batches, puree the soup using a food processor. Taste as you go along and adjust seasonings to suit your taste.

It may be served cold or hot, decorated with cilantro leaves.

Risotto along with Crimini Mushrooms and Arugula

Serving of Three (3)

Recipe

¼ pound of diced crimini mushrooms it should be cleaned and stemmed

¼ pound of diced zucchini

4 tablespoon olive oil

¼ cups wine (white)

1 finely chopped onion

1 2/3 cups uncooked long grain brown rice

4 cups low-sodium chicken broth along with water if necessary

3 tablespoon minced parsley

1 clove minced garlic

¼ cup grated parmesan cheese

Salt and pepper to taste

A lot of arugula or rocket salad

Instructions

Heat up 1 tbsp of olive oil in a big pan. Put in mushrooms and zucchini along with season, salt and pepper. Cook continuously stirring for a couple of minutes or until the zucchini and mushrooms are soften. Remove to a plate and put it aside.

With the same saucepan heat another 1 tbsp olive oil and put in the onion that is finely chopped. Sauté until onions are lucent. At this point include the uncooked rice for a couple of minutes and constantly stir. Include the wine to the mixture and cook until the wine has disappeared, this can take approximately four (4) minutes.

Include a ½ cup of broth. Allow to cook, stirring occasionally or until nearly all the broth has vanished. As this takes place include another ½ cup of broth every time the liquid is absorbed this should be done until all the broth is used and the rice is nearly cooked, if you have run out of broth use water. Add in the zucchini, mushrooms, parsley and garlic. Mix in the remaining 1 tbsp of olive oil. Include parmesan as well as salt and pepper to taste.

Move to serving plates and dress up with a lot of arugula. Serve right away.

Whole wheat Pasta and Nettle Pesto

Serving of Four (4)

Recipe

2 cups blanched young nettle leaves

4 peeled cloves of garlic

1/3 cup chopped walnuts

1/3 cup grated Parmesan cheese

1/3 cup extra-virgin olive oil

12 ounces dried whole wheat pasta

Instructions

Add together the nettle leaves walnuts and garlic in a food processor. Process and slowly add olive oil until you get to a desired evenness. Mix in the grated Parmesan cheese.

Cook pasta according to the directions on the package.

Drain pasta and place back into pot, after which stir in the nettle pesto.

Remove to a serving plate and embellish as preferred.

Tomato, Red Onion and Cucumber Salad

Recipe

2 big peeled and coarsely chopped cucumbers

3 big coarsely chopped tomatoes

2/3 cup coarsely chopped red onion

1/3 cup balsamic vinegar

½ tablespoon granulated sugar

3 tbsp extra virgin olive oil

Include salt and pepper to taste

Fresh mint leaves or basil for garnish (optional)

Instructions

In a big bowl that have a lid place all the ingredients. Cover up, and shake into mix.

flavour with salt and pepper.

Onion and Apple Soup

Serves six (6) persons

Recipe

1 Tablespoon canola oil

2 average sliced yellow onions

1 small chopped leek

½ Tablespoon fresh chopped rosemary

½ Tablespoon of fresh thyme

3 organic apples, diced into small pieces

6 cups low-sodium fat-free vegetable broth

Instructions

Heat up oil in an average sized saucepan over medium heat. Include the onions and sauté till golden brown in color.

Pour in broth and allow it to boil over average heat. Include the apples, then minimize heat to medium-low flame and allow it to simmer for ten minutes.

Salmon Salad

Servings of Four (4)

Recipe

2 large fillets, 9 ounces of wild salmon, grilled or poached then permit to chill in the fridge until cool.

1 cup halved cherry tomatoes

2 sliced red onions

1 tablespoon capers

1 tbsp fresh finely chopped dill

1 tablespoon balsamic vinegar

1 tablespoon olive oil

¼ teaspoon pepper, freshly ground

A dash of salt

Instructions

Remove skin and debone the cool salmon. Break up into chunks then add to a bowl.

Include red onion, tomatoes and capers then toss.

Combine vinegar, dill and olive oil into a minute bowl. Then add salmon chunks, once chuck has been added toss again.

Include salt and pepper to taste then refrigerate for a minimum of 30 minutes prior to serving.

Nutritious Winter Pea and Watercress Soup (Milk-Free)

Serves 6

Recipe

1 large chopped onion

1 clove of garlic

6 cups chicken or vegetable stock

1 big potato

30 ounces of frozen peas

3 ounces of watercress

Salt and pepper for tasting purpose

Instructions

Unpeel and mash garlic then put aside. Leave crushed garlic for a minimum of five to ten minutes as crushing assist in maximizing the health-protective effects.

As health-promoting composition is forming in crushed garlic, unpeel and cut up potato also chop up the large onion.

Low heat for onion and garlic so that it sweats in 2-3 tbsp of vegetable or chicken stock. Include chunks of potato and pour in the remainder of stock. Bring to a boil then simmer for about fifteen minutes or until the potato about cooked.

Put in the frozen peas then simmer for three minutes. Include the watercress and simmer for one more minute.

Take out of the heat and permit to cool for a couple of minutes. Process with a blender until it is smooth. Add salt and pepper to taste.

Tomato, Arugula and Avocado Salad

For a Serving of (4)

Ingredients

3 cups rinsed young arugula leaves

2 cups halved cherry tomatoes

1/4 cup chopped sun-dried tomatoes

2 tbsp extra-virgin olive oil

1 tbsp balsamic vinegar

2 small peeled, pitted and sliced avocados

Instructions

In a big plastic bowl that have a lid, put arugula, sun-dried tomatoes, cherry tomatoes, vinegar and olive. Toss well.

Separate then on each serving plates place the salad along with each plate serving having slices of avocado.

Carrot and Beet Salad with Ginger

One (1) Serving

Recipe

½ cup peeled and grated uncooked beets

½ cup grated organic carrots

2 tablespoon apple juice

1 tablespoon extra-virgin olive oil

½ teaspoon minced fresh ginger

1/8 teaspoon sea salt

Instructions

Add together the grated beets and carrots in a small bowl.

Combine olive oil, apple juice, ginger, and salt in a different bowl and sprinkle over salad mixture. Toss lightly and enjoy.

Spicy Tomato Soup with Basil

Serves 2

Ingredients

3 large cloves of garlic

3 ounces of peeled and sliced shallots

1 tablespoon olive oil

1 (14 ½ ozs) canned undrained stewed tomatoes

1 1/2 cups chicken broth

1/2 teaspoon apple cider vinegar

1/4 teaspoon salt

Dash of freshly red pepper (ground)

2 tablespoon chopped fresh basil

Instructions

Unpeel and crush garlic then set it aside. Leave minced garlic for a minimum 5-10 minutes after crushing to help maximize the health-protective effects.

As health-promoting composition is forming in the crushed garlic, mix shallots, chicken broth, tomatoes and apple cider vinegar in a food processor or blender until it is smooth.

Heat up olive oil in a big nonstick pot over average heat. Add in garlic at this stage then cook for around 30 seconds, constantly stir.

Include tomato assortment then bring to a boil. Remove from heat and stir the basil in.

Serve hot.

Iced Watercress and Mint Soup

Serves Four (4)

Recipe

4 large peeled and diced cucumbers

1 cup watercress

2 tbsp apple cider vinegar

1 tablespoon extra-virgin olive oil

3/4 cup fresh mint leaves, also have additional leavers for decoration

2 tablespoon fresh oregano leaves

3 tablespoon chopped fresh chives

1 ½ cups yogurt (plain)

Include salt and freshly ground pepper to taste

Instructions

Purée cucumbers in batches in a blender. Include olive oil, watercress, mint, vinegar, oregano, and chives in the blending process until smooth. Add salt and pepper to taste. Pour out soup in a bowl and mix in the yogurt. Place in the Refrigerator for two hours or until cold. Embellish with the fresh mint leaves prior to serving.

Super-Nutritious Broccoli Salad with Apples and Cranberries

Anna Gracey

Serving of six (6)

Recipe

4 cups fresh broccoli florets

½ cup cranberries (dried)

½ cup sunflower seeds

3 organic apples

1/4 cup chopped red onion

1 cup low-fat plain yoghurt with probiotic bacteria

2 Tablespoon Dijon style mustard

1/4 cup honey

Instructions

Add together the dried cranberries, broccoli florets, chopped apples, sunflower seeds and chopped onion in a big serving bowl. Then blend the plain yoghurt, honey and mustard in a small bowl.

Include dressing to the salad in the large bowl and toss. Served chilled.

Tomato, Carrot and Lentil Soup

Serving of Four (4)

Recipe

2 tablespoon extra-virgin olive oil

1 large sliced yellow onion

2 diced carrots

2 cloves of garlic

1 teaspoon ground ginger

2 teaspoon ground cumin

2 teaspoon of ground coriander seeds

1 cup lentils (red)

28 ounces or 420grams of canned tomatoes

6 cups stock vegetable

1 ½ teaspoon salt

½ teaspoon black pepper freshly ground

Serve Greek style yoghurt (optional)

Instructions

Unpeel and crush garlic then put one side. Leave minced garlic for five to ten minutes after crushing aids in maximizing its health-protective property.

As health-promoting composition is forming in the crushed garlic, heat up the olive oil in a big nonstick pot over average heat. Include onion and cook for around three (3) minutes, occasionally stirring.

Include stock, ginger, cumin, canned tomatoes, lentils, carrots, coriander, salt and pepper, then bring to boil. Cover up the pot and allow it to simmer for twenty-five (25) minutes over average heat.

Add in garlic and allow to simmer for an additional five (5) minutes.

Purée soup in batches in a blender or use an immersing hand blender to process the soup until it is smooth. Spoon the soup into bowls then top it with a generous splotch of yoghurt.

Romaine and Smoked Salmon Salad

Serving for Two (2)

Recipe

1 small head of organic romaine lettuce

5 oz smoked thinly sliced salmon

2 diced tomatoes

4 thinly sliced radishes

1 organic diagonally sliced carrot

½ peeled and diced cucumber

Half a lemon juiced

1 teaspoon freshly peeled and minced ginger root

1 tablespoon canola oil

Instructions

Place romaine lettuce on two separate plates. Top with carrots, salmon, radishes, tomatoes and cucumber.

Shake canola oil, lemon juice and minced ginger in firmly covered jar. Pour this mixture over the salad.

DESERTS

Apple Slices with Cinnamon

Serving of one (1)

Recipe

1 average sized sliced cored apple

¼ teaspoon ground cinnamon

Instructions

Put apple slices on a little serving plate then shake over with cinnamon and serve right away.

Chocolate Cake

Recipe

1 ½ cup cooked black beans

4 big eggs

1 tablespoon mint extract

1 tsp stevia

5 tablespoon canola oil

1/3 cup honey

6 tablespoon unsweetened dark cocoa powder

1 teaspoon baking powder

½ teaspoon baking soda

Pinch of salt

Fresh mint leaves, for embellishing

Instructions

Oven should be preheated to 350°Farenheit or 175°Celsius, gas 4.

Blend together beans, stevia, 2 eggs, honey, canola oil and extracted mints in a blender until it is totally smooth.

In a little bowl, mix the cocoa powder, baking powder and baking soda.

Beat the left over 2 eggs in a little bowl. Pour in the bean batter into egg mixture then mix well. Mix in cocoa powder and beat the mixture on high until it is smooth.

Scrape the batter in a greased 9" cake pan then bake for at 350 degrees Fahrenheit for around 35-45 minutes or when the toothpick comes out clean.

Chocolate Sorbet

Serving of Four (4)

Recipe

1 cup water

1 cup organic sugar (brown)

3/4 cup cocoa powder (dark)

1/8 teaspoon salt

3 oz dark chopped milk-free chocolate

1 cup rice milk

½ teaspoon vanilla extract

1/8 teaspoon xanthan gum

Instructions

Beat together sugar, water, cocoa powder and salt in a little saucepan over average heat. Bring to boil then turn off heat. Add in chocolate and whisk until chocolate is dissolved. Mix in rice milk and vanilla extract.

Transfer mixture to a blender and include xanthan gum. Process for approximately one minute.

Pour in mixture in an ice cream maker container and freeze in accordance to the manufacturer's directions.

Nettle Crepes with Raspberries

Recipe

2 organic eggs

2 cup milk that is organic

1 cup flour (all-purpose)

7 ounces lightened and chopped young nettle shoots

1 teaspoon salt

¼ teaspoon pepper (white)

Spray Vegetable cooking

Mashed fresh raspberries

Instructions

Beat eggs in an average bowl. Add milk, flour, salt, nettle and pepper, then whisk until well combined.

In a big nonstick skillet preheat over average flames. Spray with vegetable cooking.

For the initial crepe, pour around 3-4 tbsp of batter in skillet, rotate skillet quickly until the bottom is uniformly coated. Cook crepe for a minute or two or until it is golden brown. Turnover and cook the other side for an extra 30 to 60 seconds, then take away from skillet.

Do again earlier step until all the batter is gone.

Serve up crepes with raspberries that are mashed.

NB: Nettles are loaded with nitrates, and ought not to be eaten by little children, individuals with gout, or other persons that have conditions that requires a diet that is low-nitrate.

Banana Cantaloupe Smoothie

Serves Two (2)

Recipe

1 large sliced and frozen banana

1 cup seeded and coarsely chopped cantaloupe

1 cup buttermilk having probiotic bacteria

One vanilla bean seeds

1 Tablespoon honey

Instructions

Mix together all the ingredients in a food processor or blender then blend until smooth.

Decorate as preferred. Serve right away.

About The Author

Anna Gracey has always had a passion for the conditions which affect women and she has spent many years studying about Polycystic Ovary Syndrome. During Gracey's intensive research, she found that the proper diet plays an integral role in improving the symptoms of the syndrome as well as reducing resistance to insulin.

In addition, Gracey found that there are certain supplements that can be taken to improve the ovulatory function and elevate the levels of lipoprotein, which is considered to be the good type of protective cholesterol. In this book, Gracey use the knowledge she gained throughout the process of research to shine a spotlight on how to use diet to effectively manage Polycystic Ovary Syndrome.

3528314R00032

Printed in Great Britain
by Amazon.co.uk, Ltd.,
Marston Gate.